# 30 Days
# To Quit Porn

A Program for Dropping Porn Dependency

Harper Daniels

**Share your journey!**

**Let people know you're practicing mindfulness! If you'd like to share this book online, please post a picture of the cover along with #30DaysNow and #NoFap (or #NoPorn if you don't follow the *NoFap* philosophy). If you're uncomfortable sharing this mindfulness guide, you can still interact using the unique lesson hashtags. The point is to share and help others through your gained insights and growth.**

This book is meant to be a guide and does not intend to be a cure for a serious addiction. If you are experiencing a lot of pain and suffering, and believe you need medical attention, please consult a professional medical provider. Again, this book is meant to be a guide to help overcome debilitating dependencies. If the lessons and exercises in this book are followed, relief can happen. Results vary from person to person; some people may not need the entire thirty days, but it's encouraged that the entire program be read completely through at least once.

The last half of the book consists of blank note pages that the reader can use in conjunction with the exercises for each day. The note pages can be used as the reader wishes.

**Give the gift of mindfulness**. See similar guides at www.30DaysNow.com if you wish to purchase a book for a loved one. **See the disclosure below.**

### Disclosure (Shared Lessons and Exercises):

Keep in mind that our mindfulness guides share the same lessons and exercises, so there is no need to purchase more than one book; unless you are sharing with a group or giving the guides as gifts. Our mindfulness guides are created for various topics; however, they utilize the same lessons and exercises, so please be aware of this before purchasing. For example, *30 Days to Quit Porn* will mostly have the same lessons and exercises as *30 Days to Overcome Guilt* and so forth. By reading just one of our guides, you'll be able to apply the same lessons and exercises to multiple areas of your life.

Enjoy your journey of self-discovery!

# Contents

Preface...........................................................3

Day 1.........................................................6
Day 2.........................................................7
Day 3.........................................................8
Day 4.........................................................9
Day 5........................................................10
Day 6........................................................11
Day 7........................................................12
Day 8........................................................13
Day 9........................................................14
Day 10.......................................................15
Day 11.......................................................16
Day 12.......................................................17
Day 13.......................................................18
Day 14.......................................................19
Day 15.......................................................20
Day 16.......................................................21
Day 17.......................................................22
Day 18.......................................................23
Day 19.......................................................24
Day 20.......................................................25
Day 21.......................................................26
Day 22.......................................................27
Day 23.......................................................28
Day 24.......................................................29
Day 25.......................................................30
Day 26.......................................................31
Day 27.......................................................32
Day 28.......................................................33
Day 29.......................................................34
Day 30.......................................................35

Conclusion...................................................36
Note Pages...........................................Begins on 37

# Preface

The following pages involve a 30 day program made up of lessons and exercises to help you drop a porn dependency. Though these lessons and exercises can be applied to any unhealthy reliance, this program will focus specifically on the use of pornography.

For some readers, their dependency will drop quickly; and for others it'll drop gradually. In either case, if you stick with the program you'll start to witness your dependency weaken and you'll eventually drop it. Don't critique your progress throughout the program, as this isn't a competition and there isn't a goal you must attain. Let the dependency drop as you work through the exercises and lessons.

It's not necessary that you complete these days in order, nor should you be religious about completing them successfully. There is no such thing as a successful completion of this program. The bottom line is to observe and awaken, and that cannot be obtained through success, force, pressure, struggle, or competition. Simply relax, follow the program, and the dependency will drop.

You'll also notice that mindfulness, silence, and stillness are a regular discipline for each day. Because you've been influenced by a dependency based culture that demands instant gratification, silence and stillness may seem nearly impossible for you to practice. For this reason, we'll incorporate this discipline from the outset. A quiet and still mind is an incredibly powerful resource, but one that requires daily maintenance.

It should also be noted that you're not required to get rid of pornography that may be on your smartphone or computer; nor are you required to stop using porn if you're currently dependent on it. However, if you have already gone a few days without using porn, then it's advised that you continue without it. The point being: by practicing the following disciplines in the days to come, you won't even need willpower to drop the dependency; you can have porn right in front of you, and it won't have the slightest impact. Simply put, you'll drop all desire for porn without effort.

One of the most important lessons to keep in mind is to not fight the dependency or strive against it while participating in these exercises. If you find yourself using porn during the coming days, then that's completely fine as long as you stick to the program. Be careful not to develop a spirit of fighting or competition during this program – dependencies thrive on conflict.

You'll need about 15-30 minutes per day for the program; but feel free to spend more time if needed. The amount of time doesn't matter, as long as you're in an environment that allows you to concentrate without distraction.

The last portion of this book includes note pages that you can use with the exercises. It's encouraged that you write down any thoughts, insights, adaptations, lessons, mantras, etc…on those pages. The note pages can also be used to rip out and take with you. Feel free to use them as you wish.

One last thing: If you're like most people, you're dependent on caffeine, alcohol, or sugar to some extent. Do your best to lessen the consumption of these substances over the next 30 days. Can you cut consumption of these substances in half, or more? It's important that your mind is sober and your body relaxed to make the most of these exercises.

*Let people know you're practicing mindfulness! Don't forget that each exercise has a unique hashtag for online sharing.*

# Day 1

Exercise:

*Find a place without distraction, and turn off all electronics. Sit with your back straight, kneel, or lie on a hard surface (not bed) and remain in silence for 10 minutes.*

*During these 10 minutes, take deep and focused breaths and hold them for a few seconds each. Exhale slowly. Listen intently to your breathing. Don't try to change it – simply listen, and feel the air go in and out.*

*When you're ready, repeat the mantra: "**Be still. Be silent.**" Repeat this slowly multiple times out loud as well as quietly. You might experience boredom or anxiety, but continue repeating the mantra regardless. Repeat it until you're calm and ready. You can continue the deep breathing during the mantra, or take deep breaths during pauses. Don't rush.*

Each of the 30 days will have this time of silence, focused breathing, and a mantra. Except this page, the end of each day's page will remind you of the minutes you are to spend in silence and focused breathing for the day; and will also have a mantra for you to practice. You can repeat the mantras during your times of silence and focused breathing, or following. Remember, there is no right or wrong way to do this.

If you view porn today, practice the focused breathing and mantra before, during, and after viewing. Dependencies want to fight; in fact, they're energized by fighting. Instead of fighting the porn dependency, meet it with silence and observation. Let the exercises and lessons guide you.

# Day 2

Exercise:

*Ponder this question: Can you remember a time in your life when you didn't look at porn?*

Writing is extremely beneficial to the mind; especially when pondering questions. Write down your thoughts about this particular question. If your mind drifts, then write whatever thoughts emerge. It's okay if you have nothing to write, but ponder the question regardless.

Were you able to remember a period in your life when you weren't using pornography? If you're like many people in western civilization, you may have to return to memories of childhood to determine that period. It's not uncommon for a person to start using porn at an early age. Some people have viewed porn before the teenage years.

Recognize that porn dependency is a learned behavior with roots. However, it's a dependency that can be dropped quickly and completely; and you have the capability to drop it.

*10 minutes of silence and focused breathing. Repeat the mantra: "**Listen and observe.**"

# Day 3

Exercise:

*What will your next thought be?*

Try to guess what your next thought, or next two thoughts, will be.

Five minutes from now; will you be thinking about sex, work, family, a burrito, baseball, money, etc? We're not in control of our thoughts, and that scares people. We may be able to influence our thought patterns, but thoughts are more or less like clouds that come and go in a big sky. It's difficult to predict what clouds will be floating through our minds this week, let alone in five minutes.

By thinking about the question, *"What will your next thought be?"* you're allowing yourself to leave your mind for a few moments and experience thoughtlessness – which is wonderful. It's like a mental vacation.

After you've tried to answer that question, observe what thoughts actually do pop into your mind. Observe them like you would clouds in a sky. You'll witness that you're not your thoughts, which are often fantasy and not based in the present moment.

The goal of porn is to send you an endless amount of fictitious thoughts; so many that you actually believe they're part of your being. Thoughts are not real.

*10 minutes of silence and focused breathing. Repeat the mantra: **"I don't exist in fantasy. I am present. I am real."**

# Day 4

Exercise:

*Observe your body. Observe how it feels, moves, and reacts.*

Remember that most people use pornography to bring about an orgasm, or a general feeling of excitement that releases certain neurochemicals in the brain. Many people do this because they're stressed, depressed, or anxious – the world we live in can be taxing on the body, and porn offers the viewer a way to cope. That way involves manipulation of brain chemicals, often produced by the orgasm.

If you're still using pornography today, observe your body movements, sounds, sensations, and breaths during your use of it. Do your eyes look down or roll? Do you move your hands fast or slow? Is there a stopping and starting at certain intervals? Are your fingers clicking a keyboard quickly, slowly? How is your posture? Try to observe everything about your body while viewing porn. Be aware.

If you are not using porn today, then continue with the 10 minutes of silence and focused breathing, but get in touch with your body. A good way to do this is by touching each body part and saying its name, leaving your hand on the part for a few seconds and feeling its texture and warmth. Start with your head: place your hand on your head and say, *"I'm touching my head."* And then work your way down to your shoulders, arms, stomach, legs, knees, and feet. Focus your attention on one body part at a time.

*10 minutes of silence and focused breathing. Repeat the mantra: **"I am not my body."***

# Day 5

Exercise:

*On a piece of paper, write down all the labels and adjectives that you and others use to identify you.*

For example, do you see yourself as a son, daughter, mother, father, student, teacher, engineer, accountant, employee, employer, roommate, husband, wife, etc? And what adjectives do you use to label yourself; for example, do you identify yourself as failed, successful, happy, depressed, good, moral, unethical, lustful, greedy, valuable, worthless, etc? Don't only write down the labels and descriptions; but also write down what you believe others see in terms of labels and adjectives. Do you think others see you as a valuable friend, stupid student, incompetent employee, sexy girlfriend, smart person, etc?

Take as long as you need, and fill up a sheet of paper with those labels and descriptions.

After you've done that, tear the paper into multiple pieces and throw it away. Those labels and adjectives mean nothing. They're not "you." You cannot be defined, labeled, described, or controlled. What you wrote on the paper are mere words, and most people poison their conscience with such learned vocabulary. They really believe in these words – they'll even fight, stress, get sick, and die to make these words a reality. Porn, as well as most societal tools, teaches you to identify with particular words, which are only thoughts.

*10 minutes of silence and focused breathing. Repeat the mantra: "**I am not a label, title, or thought.**"

# Day 6

Exercise:

*Stand still for 5 minutes; with knees slightly bent (i.e. your legs should not be locked). At first try to remain still, but then let your body sway. Let it move any way it wishes. Feel its movement. If you're unable to stand, you can do this same exercise by extending your arm or leg from a sitting position – try to keep it straight, but then let go of trying and allow movement to happen.*

We tend to lock ourselves into particular goals, expectations, thought patters, and habits. We even go so far as to be proud of rigidity – people mistake rigidity for perseverance. This is taught to us by our culture. Everything around you may be shouting, even in a quiet whisper, that you must remain submissive and obedient.

Porn, like most dependencies, is no different in its message. It wants you to remain rigid; not to be released from its hold. If you freely moved on from porn use, it would lose you as a customer and dependent. By the way, who wants to remain rigidly dependent on something like porn for their happiness? Or I should say…false happiness.

The message of porn essentially says, "*Stay here with these images and videos. Return to them daily. Use them to your advantage. You need them for sexual fulfillment and comfort.*" Allow your body and mind to move on from porn dependency. Trust that your body and mind will sway to its own rhythm, and away from porn.

*10 minutes of silence and focused breathing. Repeat the mantra: "**I am now free to move. I am free to move on.**"

# Day 7

Exercise:

*Count to 25 slowly, pausing for a few seconds before the next number; then, count backward from 25 slowly. Try this with your eyes closed.*

Our world today is about speed. Everyone seems to be in a rush, yet most of them are unsatisfied; and, they have no clue where they're going. Chasing the next best thing is a fruitless endeavor. It's the rare person who slows down to enjoy the present moment, regardless of the nature of the moment. Because there seems to be so many problems, and most jobs are focused on resolving those problems, people are compelled to accept anxiety and rush toward a reward and conclusion. That surely isn't happiness, because happiness can only be found in the present moment, not in a hypothetical future of reward or success.

The creators of porn know this fact well, so they display the images and videos on technological platforms that allow for this constant demand to rush. How many times have you rushed through porn videos to find the one that matches your desired narrative? This is destructive to your peace of mind and health: concentration suffers, stress levels rise, and awareness to the present moment isn't possible.

It's critical to slow down. You only have one life to live – don't rush through it, and don't be dependent on anything that encourages you to rush.

*10 minutes of silence and focused breathing. Repeat the mantra: **"Slow down. Do not rush. Enjoy the present moment."**

# Day 8

Exercise:

*On a piece of paper (any size) write down the goals that you've been striving to achieve – i.e. the goals that you believe will bring you fulfillment. For example: a new job, a house in a nice neighborhood, traveling the world, a business, a family, new friends, a degree or certification, building a network, reaching a net worth of a million dollars, etc.*

*Now, tear up the paper into multiple pieces, and throw away.*

Goals can be very helpful and useful if they're not obsessed over. However, in western culture people develop a reliance on goals. Think about all the times you've said something like, *"I need to get that," "I must reach this," "I'll do anything to accomplish that"*, etc. It's often the case that people spend more time worrying about their goals, than freely doing something in the present moment to reach them. Plus, the goal in itself is fleeting, while the journey in the present moment is real and lasting.

The habit of thinking that goals must be met or else failure ensues is subtly applied to dependencies. When you've viewed porn in the past, what was the goal? What was it that you felt you needed to achieve?

*10 minutes of silence and focused breathing. Repeat the mantra: **"My happiness does not depend on meeting a goal. I'm happy now."**

# Day 9

Exercise:

*Spend 5 minutes smelling something aromatic: a piece of fruit, a spice, tea, pine, cedar, a flower, a scented candle, etc. Focus on the smell of that one thing for the entire 5 minutes. Don't let anything distract you from the smell.*

How often do you take time to enjoy a fragrant smell? One of the lies of modern society is that if you stop and enjoy your five senses too long, you'll miss out on…fill in the blank. While people are rushing toward their goals with stress levels spiking, they're totally missing out on awareness in the present moment. People stare at images of food that others have posted on the internet, but don't take the time to smell or taste food in the present moment.

What's better: watching two actors having sex in an online fantasy, or enjoying the smell of vanilla, orange, or pine in the present reality? The first is fake and illusory; the second is real and sensational. Porn does a great job from stealing time and energy from your other senses, such as smell. One of the best ways get into the present moment and away from an illusion is through focusing on smell and the use of your other senses. Don't let porn diminish your other senses any longer.

*10 minutes of silence and focused breathing. Repeat the mantra: *"I can sense the present."*

# Day 10

Exercise:

*Focus on a natural object or scene for 10 minutes, without distraction and in silence.*

Focusing on a natural object for an extended period of time is an ancient practice. How often have you stopped to observe something objectively for more than 10 minutes? When was the last time you've quietly watched a sunset, sunrise, tree sway in the wind, bird chirping, clouds passing or expanding, or just a rock? That might sound boring, but this practice is very liberating. If you look at anything long enough you start to see it from a different perspective. As easy as this exercise sounds, it's not – try it out, and see how long you can observe without thoughts impeding the practice.

Watching a bird feed may be more interesting than watching an immobile rock; but I encourage you to start with an immobile object, such as a stone or piece of wood. During this process thoughts will emerge – observe the thoughts and let them pass.

Who looks at porn as a mystic would look at a stone? Nobody does; because porn isn't natural. Porn producers don't want you to objectively see the illusion that they're actors who are uncomfortably and deceptively having sex. The purpose of porn is to hypnotize you with a false narrative; stealing your attention from the present.

*10 minutes of silence and focused breathing. Repeat the mantra: **"Be focused. Observe. Be present."***

# Day 11

Exercise:

*Imagine being a porn star in the any of the porn films that you've favored.*

Have you ever seriously considered what porn actors and actresses think and feel while on the set or in the studio? Take a moment, and put yourself in their shoes.

Imagine that a friend called you, and said, *"Hey, I have a great job for you. You'll make a thousand dollars for twelve hours of work. It's a porn shoot. We need you to fill in for someone."* Now, imagine actually saying yes, showing up to the studio, apartment, hotel room, or wherever it's being shot, and following the orders of the producer: *"Stand there," "You don't look like you're in pain. Look like you're in pain," "Stop. Stop! Change positions. Grab their head. Come on. We don't have all day," "Now scream like you're having the greatest orgasm ever," "Not like that. Do it over," "Ok everyone, we'll have to repeat this again using a different camera and angle."*

Do you think you'll be able to enjoy that work? Despite making a lot of money, would it be fun? And think of the narrative that the film is promoting: a stepfather and stepdaughter situation, a teen and teacher scenario, an unwanted gang bang, a punishment and abuse story, etc. The only person enjoying porn is the dependent viewer…and that's a fleeting enjoyment that evolves in strange ways. It's a twisted perception of reality.

*10 minutes of silence and focused breathing. Repeat the mantra: **"Fantasy is not reality. Reality is here and now."**

# Day 12

Exercise:

*If you can stand, stand on one foot and try to stay balanced as long as possible. If you're unable to stand, balance a pen on your wrist or index finger, trying not to let it fall.*

*Now let your elevated foot, or the balanced pen, drop. Don't force the drop, just let it happen naturally.*

All abnormal dependencies want you to balance them with necessary dependencies (eating, drinking, breathing, moving, sensing, etc). Porn doesn't want you to consider it abnormal or damaging to your baseline happiness. It wants you to believe that you can keep it in balance with your basic needs for survival. This is an effective lie of the dependency; and in fact, all dependencies use this lie to keep you hooked.

Understand that porn dependency doesn't help you at all; even in a balanced state. Let's say a person can balance porn with their responsibilities to care for family, work, and staying healthy. The person is fooling themselves, and the porn is slowly but surely taking from present moment awareness. It would be better if this person let the balance fail and watch porn drop to either side – that is, either completely impacting their lives negatively (many call this *hitting rock bottom*) or letting it pass away, like a dark cloud passing in a blue sky.

*10 minutes of silence and focused breathing. Repeat the mantra: *"**It is okay to let go. I can let go.**"*

# Day 13

Exercise:

*On a sheet of paper (any size) write down all the internal lies that you regularly hear about yourself – i.e. within your mind.*

*Now, tear the paper into multiple pieces, and throw away.*

It's common to have an internal voice (or voices) within your mind, playing a record of lies over and over. We eventually begin to accept these lies and let them impact our growth and happiness. Most people you see on a daily basis have these recurring internal voices; and most people are oblivious to them – sort of like white noise. This isn't a mental illness, but a way in which the mind works. We all experience these internal quiet voices whispering untruths about our being. These lies are nothing to fear, but need to be observed. Writing them down helps you observe and become aware of their deceptions.

The power of the silence, focused breathing, and mantras, which you have been practicing, is to draw out the lies. Let them manifest, and observe them. Common internal lies include: *"You are a loser," "You have become nothing, and you will never improve," "You are worthless. No one likes you," "You'll always be alone," "You're a burden,"* and so on. These thoughts are not part of you; however, the deception is to make you believe they are. Like many things in our culture, porn implants many of these lies clandestinely.

*10 minutes of silence and focused breathing. Repeat the mantra: **"Thoughts are only thoughts - nothing more."**

# Day 14

Exercise:

*For 10 minutes, look at your face in a mirror. Analyze its curvature, look closely at the color of your eyes, notice the blemishes and spots, observe its movements, etc. Look at your face as if you were observing someone else's. Do this without judgment, but observe any thoughts that emerge.*

Did you experience judgment? Were you upset? Was this an uncomfortable exercise? Were you content with the look of your face? Did any thoughts appear?

Rarely do we stop to look at our faces in a mirror for an extended period of time. You may for a quick moment while cleaning or dressing, but hardly long enough to see its uniqueness. The face may be the most important part of your body, since it's what people recognize most. However, the face that you have is not "you".

Judgment runs rampant today. Even those who say, *"I don't judge. I never judge a person"* are fooling themselves. It takes a lot of practice and mindfulness to be judgment free. It's possible to reach that awareness, but it needs to start with your perception of "you". The day you stop judging yourself, you'll stop judging others.

The hope of porn is that you will diligently judge yourself, consciously and subconsciously, so that you'll seek validation within the confines of its illusory narrative.

*10 minutes of silence and focused breathing. Repeat the mantra: **"I am not my face or body. I do not need validation."**

# Day 15

Exercise:

*Light a candle and observe its flame for 5 minutes. Watch it move and feel its heat. Appreciate its energy.*

*Now, blow out the flame.*

*(If you don't have a candle, light a match and blow it out; and if you don't have a candle or match, stare at a dim light for 5 minutes and then turn it off.)*

The temperature of a small candle flame (and match flame) is around 1200 Celsius (which is about 2000 Fahrenheit). That's a lot of energy! And within a fraction of a second, it was extinguished as you blew it out; or in the case of the light, turned off its energy source. There wasn't a gradual process with delays and stops. You blew out the highly energized flame, and that was it - from 1200 Celsius to nonexistent in no time...or should I say in present no time.

We think that our dependencies have so much energy and power. It's not just porn, but all dependencies survive on this deception of power. The truth is that dependencies don't have energy like the candle flame, though your mind may have been tricked into believing they do. The candle flame is real and powerful; whereas dependencies are illusory and fictitious.

As easily and quickly as you distinguished the flame, you can drop a dependency in the present moment.

*15 minutes of silence and focused breathing. Repeat the mantra: **"Dependency isn't real. It is extinguished."**

# Day 16

Exercise:

*Taste something by eating it very slowly for at least 5 minutes. Pick something with a lot of flavor: a piece of fruit, a strong tea, a spice, soup with many ingredients, honey, etc. Close your eyes through most of your tasting. Savor the piece of food slowly. Pay close attention to the feel of the taste on your tongue. Chew slowly.*

Porn does a great job at stealing presence away from our other senses, as does many dependencies. Since porn is directly related to our reproductive senses, the more those senses are abused the more our other senses are neglected. When was the last time you thoroughly enjoyed the taste of an orange, vanilla, dark chocolate, olive oil, or cheese? I don't mean enjoying the flavor for a few seconds and then continuing on with your meal, but to let the flavor linger before taking another bite.

The taste of a pineapple, pepper, grape, or apple is far more real and satisfying than pornography. It may sound silly to say that, but it's true, because those foods are based in reality. You can actually interact with them in the present, and they don't hypnotize you into an illusory relationship based on neurochemical reliance (the reliance I'm referring to is the orgasm that porn manipulates).

Let the taste of food bring you into the present moment.

*15 minutes of silence and focused breathing. Repeat the mantra: *"**I am free to taste.**"*

# Day 17

Exercise:

*Listen to a person intently without interruption. Only speak if the person asks you a question, but don't give a long answer. Make the conversation entirely theirs. Give them the floor, and listen to every word they are saying. Again, do not interrupt. Observe their words and facial expressions without judgment. Be patient and relaxed, even if they speak for more than a few minutes.*

Patience is a dying practice in our digital age. It appears that all business involves the perceived need to go faster, faster, and faster. Quicker responses, faster uploads, more data, rapid analysis, accelerated transportation, and all sorts of chop-chop. This false need for speed has seeped deep into our collective psyche. The western world is filled with anxiously demanding people, going nowhere fast.

This widespread lack of patience has caused a problem with regard to listening to one another. It has also caused dependency on porn to manifest extensively. People who are dependent on porn usually don't use one or two images to satisfy their cravings; they click, upload, and download multiple images or videos, and they require this action to happen at lightning speed. Practicing patience by listening intently to someone speak is a great way to slow the mind down and build meaningful relationships. The fabricated relationship of porn cannot compete with real human interaction, which requires patience.

*15 minutes of silence and focused breathing. Repeat the mantra: *"**Listen. Be patient. Listen.**"*

(22)

# Day 18

Exercise:

*Turn off your cell phone, or put it in airplane mode, for at least 1 hour, and observe the thoughts you experience. If you don't have any major responsibilities this day, or if you have all you need and don't require the phone, then turn off your cell phone for 12 hours. This exercise works best if you can go 24 hours without your cell phone activated; but go no less than 1 hour. If there are people who are immediately dependent on you, send them a text saying that you'll be unavailable, and then turn off your phone.*

Like never before in history, we live in a modern world with a plethora of distractions. These distractions fight for our attention, because money is behind the scenes. Every business is wondering how they can break your distraction from one thing so that you can be distracted by their thing – whether that thing is a product or service, such as porn. It's a constant war between everyone. Whoever can hold your attention the longest, wins the battle; but whoever can make you dependent, wins the war.

The porn industry needs for you to be distracted by its business; otherwise you might wake up to reality and enjoy the beauty of life, which includes real sex. Porn has made its way into smartphones; so no longer does the porn dependent viewer need a computer to get off. The dependent can carry porn around and access it at will, strengthening the dependency along the way.

*15 minutes of silence and focused breathing. Repeat the mantra: **"I am not distracted. I am present, here, and now."**

# Day 19

Exercise:

*Clean something slowly. Take your time; don't rush the cleaning, and be thorough. You can clean your room, car, kitchen, bathroom, bag, desk drawer, shoes...anything. Go slow, and give full attention to what you're doing. Throw away as much stuff as possible.*

Though most of us hate cleaning and only do it when the mess has become monstrous, cleaning is known to be therapeutic for a reason. We attach to our clutter fairly quickly, but we don't enjoy it. Regular cleaning is a wonderful practice because we're letting go of disorder in the present moment, in a very practical way.

Similar to a messy kitchen that can look depressing; the mind can experience depression because of pornographic clutter. Remember that porn is an illusion, so the person who utilizes porn regularly is filling the mind and body with misconceptions and fantasies that block authentic perception in the present moment. The only way to clear this type of unseemly mental clutter is through observation, understanding, and awareness.

The exercises in this book are purposed to help clear your mind from the mess that porn leaves, so you can perceive clearly. If you haven't experienced it already, waking up to a life without porn dependency is refreshing and exciting.

*15 minutes of silence and focused breathing. Repeat the mantra: *"I am clean. My mind is clear."*

# Day 20

Exercise:

*Hold a smile for 5 minutes. You don't need to do this exercise in front of a mirror; but feel free to do so if you wish. You can even do this exercise during the 15 minutes of silence and focused breathing. While holding your smile, take a moment and feel your face; actually touch the smile and the curvature of your lips and cheek bones.*

Have you ever behaved a certain way and then saw your mood change immediately? Physical exercise, such as running and weightlifting, does this for many people. Certain forms of yoga have also been used by people to change their moods. The point is: changing your behavior not only impacts other people, but can also impact your perception.

You'll notice that while you're smiling during this exercise, you may experience certain emotions. You might feel silly, embarrassed, stupid, funny, weird, or whatever. Continue smiling regardless. In fact, if you are still using porn at this point in the program, smile while you're viewing it – hold the smile until you are through with your porn use. As always, observe your thoughts while you're smiling; observe the thoughts as if they're clouds passing by in a bright blue sky.

Smiling causes an authentic reaction in our bodies and minds that is essentially good. The present moment enjoys a nice smile. So hold that smile until you no longer can.

*15 minutes of silence and focused breathing. Repeat the mantra: *"**Happiness is now. I am happy.**"

# Day 21

Exercise:

*Choose a physical symbol that will remind you to observe and be aware in the present moment. Try to choose something from nature, or that is made of natural material.*

The object you choose can be anything, but it's best if it's something that you can enjoy looking at and touching. For example, many walkers and hikers will find a unique rock small enough to carry in their hands. A stone, necklace, bracelet, seashell, cedar block, coin…anything will do, as long as you enjoy it and you can dedicate it as a tool for remembrance.

Another cunning trick of porn is to confuse the mind into forgetting you're part of the natural world. Porn requires you to use the imagination, which can be easily manipulated for the business of porn. Thus, you're taken out of physical reality. By having a symbol of remembrance, you can reconnect with the present moment. This symbol isn't meant to be an idol, god, or icon. Don't think too deeply into this. The symbol is simply a tool to help you remember where you are in the *here and now*. As long as you're aware of the present, you'll have no desire to return to the hallucination of porn.

*15 minutes of silence and focused breathing. Repeat the mantra: *"All is well. Here and now, all is well."*

# Day 22

Exercise:

*On a sheet of paper (one that you can easily save and return to later) make a list of hobbies that you've had in the past but have neglected, and also make a list of hobbies that you would like to start in the future.*

*From these lists choose one hobby from the past and one new hobby that you'd like to start. Focus only on these two – the old hobby and the new one. Make this a priority.*

How often have you said, or have heard other people say, *"I wish I had the time."* You do have the time. You just choose to think of time in the way that you've been taught to perceive it. If your life depended on it, you would certainly make the time if needed.

In fact, time is a manmade construct…don't ever forget that. There is only ever the present moment. Past and future are not here and now. We spend far too much time thinking about time. How many of your recurrent inner thoughts involve questions such as, *"When will that ever happen?"* *"When will I ever change?"* *"Why did that have to happen?"* *"If the past was different, life would be better."* These are lies that only eat into the present moment, and infect our modern world.

Porn occupies the present moment; and that moment could be used to pursue hobbies that magnify your happiness.

*15 minutes of silence and focused breathing. Repeat the mantra: **"The time is now. It is the present moment."**

# Day 23

Exercise:

*Deliberately feel the sensation of water on your skin for at least 5 minutes. You can do this exercise in the shower, while washing your hands, taking a bath, going for a swim, walking in the rain, or simply placing your hand in a sink filled with water. Close your eyes if you like.*

How often do you deliberately experience the essence of water? We take it for granted every day. It's a remarkable chemical substance in the universe that is necessary for all life. Without it, we wouldn't exist. This one transparent and fluid substance has immense capacity. A large percentage of your physical body is made of this natural substance. Experience it.

Every day we jump in the shower, wash our hands, and drink it – but rarely do we take time to slowly and deliberately appreciate our natural response to water. Porn can never give you the energy, sensation, reality, and present moment that water can give. Water is an example of a positive dependency that doesn't bind you emotionally or spiritually. Water doesn't need you; porn, however, does.

There are many lessons that water can teach: fluidity, flow, evaporation, change, motion, stillness, and life. You can't get any of those lessons through an illusion such as porn, or any unnatural dependency for that matter.

*15 minutes of silence and focused breathing. Repeat the mantra: *"I am fluid. I change. I flow."*

# Day 24

Exercise:

*Say the words "Guilt", "Shame", and "Regret" 10 times to yourself out loud. Don't rush. Pause between each repetition. For the pause, you can take a deep breath. Your eyes can remain open or closed. Again, don't rush - say the words slowly and observe any thoughts, feelings, or images that emerge internally.*

*Now, say these words again 10 times, but with a smile.*

What futile credence we give words such as Guilt, Shame and Regret. We use these words on ourselves as well as others; they become regular vocabulary for our internal recurring voices. And in the end, they're mere words that hold no power. What would these words be without a facial expression, tone, inflection, or emphasis?

When you said these three specific words, what thoughts came to mind, what did you feel, and was there a reaction in your body? If there was a reaction, such as shortness of breath or a frown, people tend to interpret it as sadness; but this reaction is a learned behavior. We've been taught to feel and think a certain way with regard to guilt, shame, and regret. The truth is: these words mean nothing.

Porn, like most dependencies, flourishes on these three words and the learned reactions they produce. But see them for that they are…mere words with no power.

*15 minutes of silence and focused breathing. Repeat the mantra: **"I am not Guilt. I am not Shame. I am not Regret."**

# Day 25

Exercise:

*On a piece of paper (any size) write down the name of your current emotion. For example, at this moment you might be feeling agitated, calm, bored, angry, anxious, excited, etc. Whatever emotion you are experiencing, give it a name and put it on paper.*

*Now, write down "I'm experiencing this emotion in the present moment and it will pass. It's only an emotion."*

*You can throw the paper away, or hold onto it if you wish.*

Similar to how we give certain words credence, we tend to give our emotions a lot of trust. We also tend to blame the outside world for emotions we are feeling: "*They made me angry*," "*I'm depressed because they didn't want me*," "*If they gave me the job, I would be happy.*"

The emotions you feel are in you, not in the outer world. No one can cause you to feel or emote in a particular way; if they're able to, it's only because you let them. A great way to let a harmful emotion pass is to observe it; and a good start is by giving it a name and seeing it as powerless.

It's commonplace to blame others for our pain. Instead of seeing the emotion for what it is and letting it pass, we've been taught to rely on dependencies, like porn, to manage the emotional reaction. Wake up! Emotions are not you.

*15 minutes of silence and focused breathing. Repeat the mantra: "**I am not an emotion. All emotions that I experience will pass.**"

(30)

# Day 26

(Share this experience using #30DaysBlue)

Exercise:

*Today, look for the color blue in your surrounding environment. If possible, spend the entire day looking for the color blue in the places you go. Whether you're doing this exercise in a bedroom, office, classroom, outside, or while traveling, look for the color blue in all things that surround you. If you think you'll forget to do this throughout the entire day, spend at least 20 focused minutes practicing this exercise at some point.*

Focused attention is something that must be practiced - it doesn't come easy in our rapid paced society. Instead of encouraging us to focus and observe, the modern world encourages us to rush and get things done.

Searching for a color or shape helps to slow down our accelerated and cyclical thought patterns, and reminds us that there's more to the world than the chaotic thoughts we collectively and daily experience. By searching for the color blue, your mind can escape the fictitious grip of anxiety, lust, desire, depression, worry, fear, or any other potent emotion. When you were using porn, were you aware of the colors in the film or image? Most likely not.

Porn functions to distract your conscience from present reality. Look for the color blue today, and wake up to life in the present moment.

*15 minutes of silence and focused breathing. Repeat the mantra: *"I am focused, here and now."*

# Day 27

Exercise:

*Make yourself laugh for 5 minutes. Don't stop laughing. You might feel strange, weird, embarrassed, or stupid…it doesn't matter, just laugh. Try to laugh alone and without the aid of a comedy or joke. If you don't know how to start, just start making the noises that typically accompany your laughter.*

What feelings did you experience during this exercise? Many people report feeling embarrassed or goofy, which is great; however, most people also report a feeling of relief and buoyancy when they've completed this exercise.

Similar to holding a smile, laughing for 5 minutes is a fantastic way to come into present awareness. If you think about it, humor is necessary for life. How sad is the person who is unable to laugh at the experiences of life? After all, life is funny.

If you ever experience the desire to use porn again, simply laugh at it. Consider how porn is idiotic and frivolous; it really is a funny dependency. No other living thing on the planet becomes dependent on watching naked bodies bang for bucks. It's quite stupid, and thus funny. If you perceive porn for what it truly is - a fictitious, impractical, and frivolous imagery – then it can be easily dropped.

*15 minutes of silence and focused breathing. Repeat the mantra: *"**Life is wonderful, funny, and real.**"*

# Day 28

Exercise:

*Look at a picture or painting for 10 minutes, alone, in silence, and without any distraction. It would be best if the picture isn't of family or friends, but it could have been created by someone you know. Try to choose a work of art for this exercise, but any picture or painting will suffice.*

Porn isn't art; though some people will argue it is – those people are typically arguing in order to hold onto the dependency. Porn producers, directors, and actors aren't making pornography for the purpose of art; instead, they're making it to capitalize off peoples' dependencies. Despite porn being image based, have you ever seen porn advertised as art?

When images of pornography occupy the mind, there's a loss of connection to images that can be helpful to the awakened mind. The purpose of this exercise is to return the mind to an appreciation of truly inventive and innovative art. A printed picture hanging in a cheap motel room has more artistry than the most popular trending porn film.

Observing a picture, photo, or print for an extended period of time can aid the mind in slowing down. You may have had a photo of a landscape hanging in your home for many years, but have you ever taken the time to carefully analyze it? Take some time and do that. Appreciate the image, and observe your thoughts in the process.

*15 minutes of silence and focused breathing. Repeat the mantra: "**Stillness. Silence. Peace. Presence.**"*

# Day 29

Exercise:

*Go for a mindfulness walk for at least 10 minutes. Focus on each step. Feel the steps: the feel of your feet hitting the ground, your heel rolling forward, your toes, the bend of your knees, your hips working to balance your posture, the swinging of your arms, etc. Don't rush; go slow. Focus on your breathing as well. Get in tune with your body as you step. Pay attention to your physical senses throughout the walk. Focus – don't listen to music or be distracted.*

Human beings have always used walking as a natural therapeutic exercise. There is something about walking, and focusing on the walk, that calms the mind and soul. The longer one walks, the more relaxed the person feels.

Any moment is a good time to walk and experience your inner and outer environment. During long walks, thoughts will emerge that will allow you to graciously observe them. Let the thoughts pass; you may even have emotions that emerge, observe those and let them pass as well. Focusing on your steps will help you clear the mind of clutter. Walking in the early morning and at dusk is especially beneficial.

A 20 minute walk brings more comfort, stillness, peace, focus, and awareness than thousands of hours of using porn. Walk every day, as much as you can.

*15 minutes of silence and focused breathing. Repeat the mantra: *"I am relaxed. I am at peace."*

# Day 30

Exercise:

*One last time, take a piece of paper (one that you can keep) and write down all that you are grateful for – these things don't have to be in any particular order of importance.*

*Next to each thing you list, write "Thank you."*

Strong dependencies don't encourage gratitude. The person who isn't thankful for all that life gives is typically quite miserable, and dependencies flourish on that misery. The truly grateful person can let go at any time. A thankful person is a happy person.

Have you ever heard anyone say, *"I'm so grateful for porn! I wrote a letter to the producer of my favorite film, thanking him for his hard work. I also contacted the actors and marketers and thanked them for benefiting my life."* Nobody is thankful for porn; which is a clear sign that it's a destructive dependency.

Not only is it unhealthy, but porn doesn't encourage a grateful mind and soul. With only one life to live in the present moment, it's important to always emphasize a grateful heart. Spend time with people who are grateful, and do things that encourage a thankful heart. Anything that causes misery and depression, such as porn use, isn't worth giving attention to.

*15 minutes of silence and focused breathing. Repeat the mantra: **"I am grateful. I am thankful."**

# Conclusion

If you've made it through the 30 days, that's wonderful! Whether you sense it or not, you have developed some amazing skills that you can carry into other areas of your life. All that we experience is in the present moment, and to be reliant on an unhealthy dependency isn't a good use of the present. Hopefully you've dropped your dependency and moved on to more valuable experiences.

If there were any particular exercises, lessons, and mantras that helped you the most, pay close attention to those. I encourage you to continually practice the ones that have been most beneficial to you. I also want to encourage you to modify the exercises as well as create your own, tailored to your present experience. No two people are the same. As you grow into awareness and free from dependency, your practices will evolve and you'll gain liberation.

Enjoy freedom from porn dependency, and don't bother looking back. Stay grounded in the present moment.

# *Notes for Day 1*

(Use this page to write down thoughts, reminders, ideas, prayers, mantras, revelations, lessons, modifications to the exercise, or experiences. If you'd like to share something, please post using **#30DaysNow** or use the exercise's unique hashtag.)

_____

_____

_____

_____

_____

_____

_____

_____

_____

_____

_____

_____

_____

_____

_____

_____

_____

_____

_____

_____

_____

_____

_____

_____

_____

_____

_____

_____

# Notes for Day 2

(Use this page to write down thoughts, reminders, ideas, prayers, mantras, revelations, lessons, modifications to the exercise, or experiences. If you'd like to share something, please post using **#30DaysNow** or use the exercise's unique hashtag.)

# *Notes for Day 3*

(Use this page to write down thoughts, reminders, ideas, prayers, mantras, revelations, lessons, modifications to the exercise, or experiences. If you'd like to share something, please post using **#30DaysNow** or use the exercise's unique hashtag.)

# *Notes for Day 4*

(Use this page to write down thoughts, reminders, ideas, prayers, mantras, revelations, lessons, modifications to the exercise, or experiences. If you'd like to share something, please post using **#30DaysNow** or use the exercise's unique hashtag.)

# *Notes for Day 5*

(Use this page to write down thoughts, reminders, ideas, prayers, mantras, revelations, lessons, modifications to the exercise, or experiences. If you'd like to share something, please post using **#30DaysNow** or use the exercise's unique hashtag.)

# *Notes for Day 6*

(Use this page to write down thoughts, reminders, ideas, prayers, mantras, revelations, lessons, modifications to the exercise, or experiences. If you'd like to share something, please post using **#30DaysNow** or use the exercise's unique hashtag.)

# *Notes for Day 7*

(Use this page to write down thoughts, reminders, ideas, prayers, mantras, revelations, lessons, modifications to the exercise, or experiences. If you'd like to share something, please post using **#30DaysNow** or use the exercise's unique hashtag.)

# *Notes for Day 8*

(Use this page to write down thoughts, reminders, ideas, prayers, mantras, revelations, lessons, modifications to the exercise, or experiences. If you'd like to share something, please post using **#30DaysNow** or use the exercise's unique hashtag.)

_____

_____

_____

_____

_____

_____

_____

_____

_____

_____

_____

_____

_____

_____

_____

_____

_____

_____

_____

_____

_____

_____

_____

_____

_____

_____

_____

# *Notes for Day 9*

(Use this page to write down thoughts, reminders, ideas, prayers, mantras, revelations, lessons, modifications to the exercise, or experiences. If you'd like to share something, please post using **#30DaysNow** or use the exercise's unique hashtag.)

# *Notes for Day 10*

(Use this page to write down thoughts, reminders, ideas, prayers, mantras, revelations, lessons, modifications to the exercise, or experiences. If you'd like to share something, please post using **#30DaysNow** or use the exercise's unique hashtag.)

# *Notes for Day 11*

(Use this page to write down thoughts, reminders, ideas, prayers, mantras, revelations, lessons, modifications to the exercise, or experiences. If you'd like to share something, please post using **#30DaysNow** or use the exercise's unique hashtag.)

_____

_____

_____

_____

_____

_____

_____

_____

_____

_____

_____

_____

_____

_____

_____

_____

_____

_____

_____

_____

_____

_____

_____

_____

_____

_____

_____

_____

_____

# *Notes for Day 12*

(Use this page to write down thoughts, reminders, ideas, prayers, mantras, revelations, lessons, modifications to the exercise, or experiences. If you'd like to share something, please post using **#30DaysNow** or use the exercise's unique hashtag.)

# *Notes for Day 13*

(Use this page to write down thoughts, reminders, ideas, prayers, mantras, revelations, lessons, modifications to the exercise, or experiences. If you'd like to share something, please post using **#30DaysNow** or use the exercise's unique hashtag.)

_____
_____
_____
_____
_____
_____
_____
_____
_____
_____
_____
_____
_____
_____
_____
_____
_____
_____
_____
_____
_____
_____
_____
_____
_____
_____
_____

# *Notes for Day 14*

(Use this page to write down thoughts, reminders, ideas, prayers, mantras, revelations, lessons, modifications to the exercise, or experiences. If you'd like to share something, please post using **#30DaysNow** or use the exercise's unique hashtag.)

# *Notes for Day 15*

(Use this page to write down thoughts, reminders, ideas, prayers, mantras, revelations, lessons, modifications to the exercise, or experiences. If you'd like to share something, please post using **#30DaysNow** or use the exercise's unique hashtag.)

# *Notes for Day 16*

(Use this page to write down thoughts, reminders, ideas, prayers, mantras, revelations, lessons, modifications to the exercise, or experiences. If you'd like to share something, please post using **#30DaysNow** or use the exercise's unique hashtag.)

# *Notes for Day 17*

(Use this page to write down thoughts, reminders, ideas, prayers, mantras, revelations, lessons, modifications to the exercise, or experiences. If you'd like to share something, please post using **#30DaysNow** or use the exercise's unique hashtag.)

# Notes for Day 18

(Use this page to write down thoughts, reminders, ideas, prayers, mantras, revelations, lessons, modifications to the exercise, or experiences. If you'd like to share something, please post using **#30DaysNow** or use the exercise's unique hashtag.)

# *Notes for Day 19*

(Use this page to write down thoughts, reminders, ideas, prayers, mantras, revelations, lessons, modifications to the exercise, or experiences. If you'd like to share something, please post using **#30DaysNow** or use the exercise's unique hashtag.)

# *Notes for Day 20*

(Use this page to write down thoughts, reminders, ideas, prayers, mantras, revelations, lessons, modifications to the exercise, or experiences. If you'd like to share something, please post using **#30DaysNow** or use the exercise's unique hashtag.)

# *Notes for Day 21*

(Use this page to write down thoughts, reminders, ideas, prayers, mantras, revelations, lessons, modifications to the exercise, or experiences. If you'd like to share something, please post using **#30DaysNow** or use the exercise's unique hashtag.)

_____

_____

_____

_____

_____

_____

_____

_____

_____

_____

_____

_____

_____

_____

_____

_____

_____

_____

_____

_____

_____

_____

_____

_____

_____

_____

# Notes for Day 22

(Use this page to write down thoughts, reminders, ideas, prayers, mantras, revelations, lessons, modifications to the exercise, or experiences. If you'd like to share something, please post using **#30DaysNow** or use the exercise's unique hashtag.)

# *Notes for Day 23*

(Use this page to write down thoughts, reminders, ideas, prayers, mantras, revelations, lessons, modifications to the exercise, or experiences. If you'd like to share something, please post using **#30DaysNow** or use the exercise's unique hashtag.)

_____

_____

_____

_____

_____

_____

_____

_____

_____

_____

_____

_____

_____

_____

_____

_____

_____

_____

_____

_____

_____

_____

_____

_____

_____

# *Notes for Day 24*

(Use this page to write down thoughts, reminders, ideas, prayers, mantras, revelations, lessons, modifications to the exercise, or experiences. If you'd like to share something, please post using **#30DaysNow** or use the exercise's unique hashtag.)

# *Notes for Day 25*

(Use this page to write down thoughts, reminders, ideas, prayers, mantras, revelations, lessons, modifications to the exercise, or experiences. If you'd like to share something, please post using **#30DaysNow** or use the exercise's unique hashtag.)

# *Notes for Day 26*

(Use this page to write down thoughts, reminders, ideas, prayers, mantras, revelations, lessons, modifications to the exercise, or experiences. If you'd like to share online, please post using **#30DaysNow** or use the exercise's unique hashtag.)

# Notes for Day 27

(Use this page to write down thoughts, reminders, ideas, prayers, mantras, revelations, lessons, modifications to the exercise, or experiences. If you'd like to share something, please post using **#30DaysNow** or use the exercise's unique hashtag.)

# *Notes for Day 28*

(Use this page to write down thoughts, reminders, ideas, prayers, mantras, revelations, lessons, modifications to the exercise, or experiences. If you'd like to share something, please post using **#30DaysNow** or use the exercise's unique hashtag.)

# *Notes for Day 29*

(Use this page to write down thoughts, reminders, ideas, prayers, mantras, revelations, lessons, modifications to the exercise, or experiences. If you'd like to share something, please post using **#30DaysNow** or use the exercise's unique hashtag.)

_____

_____

_____

_____

_____

_____

_____

_____

_____

_____

_____

_____

_____

_____

_____

_____

_____

_____

_____

_____

_____

_____

_____

_____

_____

# *Notes for Day 30*

(Use this page to write down thoughts, reminders, ideas, prayers, mantras, revelations, lessons, modifications to the exercise, or experiences. If you'd like to share something, please post using **#30DaysNow** or use the exercise's unique hashtag.)

To be mindful is to experience life in the present moment...it's the only moment we have.

*Don't forget to leave an online review.*

*Thank you!*

www.ingramcontent.com/pod-product-compliance
Lightning Source LLC
Chambersburg PA
CBHW031250280526
45784CB00004B/1798